CROHN'S DISEASE DIET COOKBOOK

200+ Nutritional Recipes to Relieve the Symptoms of Crohn's Disease & A Comprehensive Strategies to Manage IBD with 28 Days Meal Plan

EDWARD LINDA

Table of Contents

INTRODUCTION

Crohn's disease is a lifelong condition that causes inflammation and irritation along parts of the digestive tract. Like ulcerative colitis, Crohn's is an inflammatory bowel disease (IBD). During a flare-up, a person may benefit from eating soft, bland, sufficiently nutritious foods.

It may also be best to avoid foods that trigger inflammation. In this article, we describe the symptoms of a Crohn's disease flare-up and explain the best foods to eat during one. We also look at which foods it is best to avoid during a flare-up.

Crohn's disease is a perplexing and persistent autoimmune disorder that fundamentally targets the digestive system. This condition has perplexed medical professionals and patients alike due to its multifaceted and enigmatic nature. It can manifest anywhere along the gastrointestinal tract, leading to an array of debilitating symptoms. These symptoms include severe abdominal pain, prolonged diarrhea, unexplained weight loss, fatigue, and more.

Definition of Crohn's Disease

Crohn's disease is a type of inflammatory bowel disease (IBD). It causes swelling of the tissues (inflammation) in your digestive tract, which can lead to abdominal pain, severe diarrhea, fatigue, weight loss and malnutrition.
Inflammation caused by Crohn's disease can involve different areas of the digestive tract in different people,

most commonly the small intestine. This inflammation often spreads into the deeper layers of the bowel. Crohn's disease can be both painful and debilitating, and sometimes may lead to life-threatening complications.

There's no known cure for Crohn's disease, but therapies can greatly reduce its signs and symptoms and even bring about long-term remission and healing of inflammation. With treatment, many people with Crohn's disease are able to function well.

Low residue diet

During a Crohn's flare-up, a doctor may recommend a person follow a low residue diet. This can help the bowels rest.
A Crohn's flare-up can trigger or worsen symptoms such as:
• diarrhea
• bloating
• abdominal pain and cramping
• nausea
• loss of appetite
Diarrhea and an ongoing lack of appetite can lead to dehydration and malnutrition.
If a flare-up is severe, a doctor may recommend a liquid diet, a feeding tube, or intravenous (IV) nutrition.
The rest of this article will explore how certain foods and drinks affect Crohn's symptoms during a flare-up.

Refined grains

Studies suggest certain insoluble fibers can worsen IBD symptoms during a flare-up because they are more difficult to digest. As refined grains have less insoluble fiber than whole grains, they tend to pass more quickly and easily through the digestive tract.
Examples of refined grains include:
• white bread
• white rice
• pasta
• plain crackers
• rice snacks

Low fiber fruits

Low fiber fruits are easy on the digestive system while containing various nutrients.
Examples include:
• bananas
• honeydew melon
• watermelon
• cantaloupe
• peaches
The amount of fiber in a piece of fruit changes as it ripens.
Ripe fruits generally have less fiber
than unripe fruits.

Fruit preparation

Removing the skin or peel from a piece of fruit can reduce its content of insoluble fibers such as lignin and cellulose. Cooking fruits can soften them, making them easier to digest. Canned fruits are a convenient fruit option for people experiencing a Crohn's flare.

However, they can also contain large amounts of added sugar. To reduce added sugar intake, people can choose fruits canned in juice instead of syrup. While these preparations can make it easier for the gut to tolerate fruit, people experiencing a Crohn's flare should still eat them only in moderation, as excess consumption may trigger symptoms.

Lean proteins

Protein is a critical part of a balanced diet and essential for overall health. However, many animal protein sources are also high in dietary fats. A high intake of animal fats is a risk factor for developing IBD. Consuming high levels of dietary fat can also worsen existing IBD symptoms. Prioritizing lean protein sources can help a person maintain adequate nutrition while minimizing the risk of IBD symptoms.

Lean meats

Skinless chicken and turkey are good examples of lean meats. When purchasing red meat, such as pork, it is best to select the leanest cut available and trim any visible excess fat. Experts recommend that people experiencing a Crohn's flare-up cook proteins to a soft texture and avoid tough or chewy meat cuts. Doing so can reduce the burden these foods place on the digestive process.

Eggs

Eggs are excellent sources of lean protein. Egg yolks also contain large amounts of vitamin A and vitamin D. People with Crohn's often have deficiencies of these two vitamins.

Soy products

In addition to lean protein, soy products such as tofu contain bioactive peptides.
Some animal research also suggests that they have antioxidant and anti-inflammatory properties, which may help manage IBD.

Oily fish

Not all fats have a negative effect on people with IBD. Oily fish contain healthy fats, including omega-3 fatty acids. These fight inflammation and may help reduce the risk of heart disease and certain cancers.
Health experts often recommend eating at least two servings of oily fish per week. These include trout, salmon, mackerel, herring, tuna, and sardines.

Yogurt and other dairy products

Many yogurts contain probiotics, which are healthy bacteria that may help reduce inflammation in the gut. However, some research suggests there is not yet enough evidence to understand whether probiotics are truly effective in helping to manage Crohn's disease. Other dairy products, such as milk and cheese, can be rich in calcium. Manufacturers may also fortify them with vitamin A.

However, many contain lactose, a type of sugar. Some doctors recommend people with Crohn's try eliminating lactose from their diet, as it can trigger digestive discomfort in people with an intolerance.

Drinks

Still drinks can help people stay hydrated and increase their nutritional intake without irritating the stomach.

Juices

Many vegetable and fruit juices are low in fiber and contain high levels of vitamins and minerals. Manufacturers may fortify some products with additional nutrients.
Although it is best to avoid consuming too much sugar during a Crohn's flare-up, a daily glass of diluted fruit juice that contains no added sugar can help boost a person's nutrient intake as part of a varied diet.
Vitamin C from fruit juice can also help the gut absorb iron.

Protein shakes and meal replacements

Sometimes people cannot tolerate any solid foods during a Crohn's flare. In these cases, doctors may recommend following a liquid diet. Protein shakes are the best way to maximize calories and protein on a liquid diet. Choosing a protein shake that is low in added sugars is important.

Symptoms

In Crohn's disease, any part of your small or large intestine can be involved. It may involve multiple segments, or it may be continuous. In some people, the disease is only in the colon, which is part of the large intestine. Signs and symptoms of Crohn's disease can range from mild to severe. They usually develop gradually, but sometimes will come on suddenly, without warning. You may also have periods of time when you have no signs or symptoms (remission).

When the disease is active, symptoms typically include:
• Diarrhea
• Fever
• Fatigue
• Abdominal pain and cramping
• Blood in your stool
• Mouth sores
• Reduced appetite and weight loss
• Pain or drainage near or around the anus due to inflammation from a tunnel into the skin (fistula)

Other signs and symptoms

People with severe Crohn's disease may also experience symptoms outside of the intestinal tract, including:
• Inflammation of skin, eyes and joints
• Inflammation of the liver or bile ducts
• Kidney stones
• Iron deficiency (anemia)
• Delayed growth or sexual development, in children

Stages of Crohn's Disease

Crohn's disease often gets worse over time. An endoscopy can show your doctor how much inflammation you have in your intestines. That, along with your symptoms, helps them know how advanced your Crohn's disease is.

Mild Crohn's disease

People with mild Crohn's disease have symptoms like diarrhea, but they don't have:
• Fever
• Major weight loss
• Signs of infection or blockages in their intestines

Moderate to severe Crohn's disease

Along with diarrhea and abdominal pain or tenderness, you could have:
• Fever
• Nausea or vomiting
• Noticeable weight loss

Severe Crohn's disease

This stage may bring:
• Blockages or infections in your intestines
• Symptoms that don't respond to treatment
• Symptoms in places other than your digestive tract, such as your skin, eyes, joints, liver, and kidneys

Diagnosis of Crohn's disease

Diagnosing Crohn's disease typically involves a combination of clinical evaluation, medical tests, and procedures. Here is an overview of the diagnostic process:
• Medical History and Physical Examination: The first step is a thorough review of the patient's medical history, including their symptoms and family history of digestive disorders. A physical examination helps identify signs of inflammation and abdominal tenderness.

• Blood Tests: Blood tests may be conducted to check for signs of inflammation and to rule out other conditions that can mimic Crohn's disease.

• Imaging Studies: Various imaging techniques can be used to visualize the gastrointestinal tract. These include:

• Colonoscopy: A flexible, lighted tube with a camera is inserted through the rectum to examine the colon and the end of the small intestine.

• Upper Endoscopy: This involves a similar procedure but examines the upper part of the digestive tract, including the esophagus and stomach.

• Capsule Endoscopy: The patient swallows a small camera-containing capsule that takes pictures of the entire small intestine.

• X-rays and CT Scans: These can provide detailed images of the digestive tract and help identify areas of inflammation, strictures, or fistulas.

• Biopsy: During endoscopy, the doctor may take tissue samples (biopsies) from the affected areas to confirm the presence of inflammation characteristic of Crohn's disease.

• Stool Tests: Stool samples may be analyzed to rule out infections and to assess for signs of gastrointestinal bleeding or inflammation.

• Diagnostic Criteria: Diagnosis is often based on a combination of clinical, imaging, and laboratory findings. It should meet established criteria for Crohn's disease, including the pattern, location, and depth of inflammation.

The diagnosis of Crohn's disease can be challenging, as its symptoms can mimic other gastrointestinal conditions. Once diagnosed, treatment options can range from medications to lifestyle changes and, in severe cases, surgical interventions to manage the disease and improve the patient's quality of life. A comprehensive approach involving gastroenterologists, radiologists, and pathologists is typically needed to reach an accurate diagnosis.

Crohn's Disease Treatment

There's no single treatment that's right for everyone with Crohn's disease. Your treatment will depend on what's causing your symptoms and how serious they are. Your doctor will try to reduce the inflammation in your digestive tract and keep you from having complications.

Medications for Crohn's disease

Crohn's disease is mostly treated with medications, including:
• Anti-inflammatory drugs. Examples include mesalamine (Asacol, Lialda, Pentasa), olsalazine (Dipentum), and sulfasalazine (Azulfidine). Side effects include upset stomach, headache, nausea, diarrhea, and rash. These medicines are used only in mild cases.
• Corticosteroids, a more powerful type of anti-inflammatory drug. Examples include budesonide (Entocort) and prednisone or methylprednisolone (Solu-Medrol). If you take these for a long time, side effects can be serious and may include bone thinning, muscle loss, skin problems, and a higher risk of infection.
• Immune system modifiers (immunomodulators), such as azathioprine (Imuran, Azasan) and methotrexate (Rheumatrex, Trexall). It can take up to 6 months for these drugs to work. They also bring a higher risk of infections that could be life-threatening.

• Antibiotics such as ciprofloxacin (Cipro) and metronidazole (Flagyl) to fight infections in your digestive system caused by Crohn's disease. Metronidazole can cause a metallic taste in your mouth, nausea, and tingling, or numbness of your hands and feet. Ciprofloxacin can cause nausea and tears in your Achilles tendon.
• Drugs for diarrhea including loperamide in small doses.

Biologic medicines may be included in your treatment if you have moderate to severe Crohn's disease. The anti-tumor necrosis factor drugs are often the first choice and include:
• Adalimumab (Humira)
• Adalimumab-atto (Amjevita)
• Certolizumab pegol (Cimzia)
• Infliximab (Remicade)
• Infliximab-abda (Renflexis)
• Infliximab-dyyb (Inflectra)
• Infliximab-axxq (Avsola)
Other biologics approved for Crohn's disease include:
• Natalizumab (Tysabri)
• Risankizumab-rzaa (Skyrizi)
• Ustekinumab (Stelara)
• Vedolizumab (Entyvio)
Once you start treatment, your doctor will check back in several weeks to see how well it works. You'll continue treatment until you reach remission (when your symptoms ease). When that happens, your doctor may prescribe "maintenance therapy" to keep your symptoms at bay. If you don't get better, you'll need stronger treatment. Your doctor may suggest nutritional supplements , too.

Complementary and alternative treatment options for Crohn's disease

When you use nonmedical treatment options instead of medical ones, they're called alternative therapies. Those used along with medical treatments are called complementary therapies.

Medication is the main treatment for Crohn's disease, but many people use complementary therapies to help ease symptoms. They include:
• Mind-body therapies such as relaxation, meditation, hypnosis, acupuncture, yoga, and exercise
• Dietary supplements like omega-3 fatty acids and curcumin
• Probiotics, foods, or supplements containing microorganisms that boost "good" bacteria in your gut
• Medical cannabis

Home remedies for Crohn's disease

Some things you can do on your own may also help relieve your Crohn's symptoms.
• Avoid NSAIDs. Use acetaminophen instead.
• Quit smoking. This may help reduce flare-ups, lessen the amount of medication you need, and lower your chances of surgery.
• Manage stress. Stress doesn't cause Crohn's disease, but it can make symptoms worse. Try some of the mind-body therapies above, such as meditation or yoga.

When to see a doctor

See your doctor if you have persistent changes in your bowel habits or if you have any of the signs and symptoms of Crohn's disease, such as:
• Abdominal pain
• Blood in your stool
• Nausea and vomiting
• Diarrhea lasting more than two weeks
• Unexplained weight loss
• Fever in addition to any of the above symptoms

Types of Crohn's Disease

There are five types of Crohn's, based on which part of your digestive tract is affected.
• Ileocolitis, the most common form of Crohn's disease, involves your colon and the last part of your small intestine (called the ileum or terminal ileum).
• Crohn's colitis or granulomatous colitis affects only your colon.
• Gastroduodenal Crohn's disease affects your stomach and the first part of your small intestine (called the duodenum).
• Ileitis affects your ileum.
• Jejunoileitis causes small areas of inflammation in the upper half of your small intestine (called the jejunum).

Causes

The exact cause of Crohn's disease remains unknown. Previously, diet and stress were suspected, but now doctors know that these factors may aggravate, but don't cause, Crohn's disease. Several factors likely play a role in its development.

• Immune system. It's possible that a virus or bacterium may trigger Crohn's disease; however, scientists have yet to identify such a trigger. When your immune system tries to fight off an invading microorganism or environmental triggers, an atypical immune response causes the immune system to attack the cells in the digestive tract, too.

• Heredity. Crohn's disease is more common in people who have family members with the disease, so genes may play a role in making people more likely to have it. However, most people with Crohn's disease do not have a family history of the disease.

Risk factors

Risk factors for Crohn's disease may include:

• Age. Crohn's disease can occur at any age, but you're likely to develop the condition when you're young. Most people who develop Crohn's disease are diagnosed before they're around 30 years old.

• Ethnicity. Although Crohn's disease can affect any ethnic group, whites have the highest risk, especially people of Eastern European (Ashkenazi) Jewish descent. However, the incidence of Crohn's disease is increasing among Black people who live in North America and the United Kingdom. Crohn's disease is also being increasingly seen in the Middle Eastern population and among migrants to the United States.

• Family history. You're at higher risk if you have a first-degree relative, such as a parent, sibling or child, with the disease. As many as 1 in 5 people with Crohn's disease has a family member with the disease.

• Cigarette smoking. Cigarette smoking is the most important controllable risk factor for developing Crohn's disease. Smoking also leads to more-severe disease and a greater risk of having surgery. If you smoke, it's important to stop.

• Nonsteroidal anti-inflammatory medications. These include ibuprofen (Advil, Motrin IB, others), naproxen sodium (Aleve), diclofenac sodium and others. While they do not cause Crohn's disease, they can lead to inflammation of the bowel that makes Crohn's disease worse.

Complications

Crohn's disease may lead to one or more of the following complications:

• Bowel obstruction. Crohn's disease can affect the entire thickness of the intestinal wall. Over time, parts of the bowel can scar and narrow, which may block the flow of digestive contents, often known as a stricture. You may require surgery to widen the stricture or sometimes to remove the diseased portion of your bowel.

• Ulcers. Chronic inflammation can lead to open sores (ulcers) anywhere in your digestive tract, including your mouth and anus, and in the genital area (perineum).

• Fistulas. Sometimes ulcers can extend completely through the intestinal wall, creating a fistula — an abnormal connection between different body parts. Fistulas can develop between your intestine and your skin, or between your intestine and another organ. Fistulas near or around the anal area (perianal) are the most common kind. When fistulas develop inside the abdomen, it may lead to infections and abscesses, which are collections of pus. These can be life-threatening if not treated. Fistulas may form between loops of bowel, in the bladder or vagina, or through the skin, causing continuous drainage of bowel contents to your skin.

• Anal fissure. This is a small tear in the tissue that lines the anus or in the skin around the anus where infections can occur. It's often associated with painful bowel movements and may lead to a perianal fistula.

• Malnutrition. Diarrhea, abdominal pain and cramping may make it difficult for you to eat or for your intestine to absorb enough nutrients to keep you nourished. It's also common to develop anemia due to low iron or vitamin B-12 caused by the disease.

• Colon cancer. Having Crohn's disease that affects your colon increases your risk of colon cancer. General colon cancer screening guidelines for people without Crohn's disease call for a colonoscopy at least every 10 years beginning at age 45. In people with Crohn's disease affecting a large part of the colon, a colonoscopy to screen for colon cancer is recommended about 8 years after disease onset and generally is performed every 1 to 2 years afterward. Ask your doctor whether you need to have this test done sooner and more frequently.

• Skin disorders. Many people with Crohn's disease may also develop a condition called hidradenitis suppurativa. This skin disorder involves deep nodules, tunnels and abscesses in the armpits, groin, under the breasts, and in the perianal or genital area.

• Other health problems. Crohn's disease can also cause problems in other parts of the body. Among these problems are low iron (anemia), osteoporosis, arthritis, and gallbladder or liver disease.

• Medication risks. Certain Crohn's disease drugs that act by blocking functions of the immune system are associated with a small risk of developing cancers such as lymphoma and skin cancers. They also increase the risk of infections.Corticosteroids can be associated with a risk of osteoporosis, bone fractures, cataracts, glaucoma, diabetes and high blood pressure, among other conditions. Work with your doctor to determine risks and benefits of medications.

• Blood clots. Crohn's disease increases the risk of blood clots in veins and arteries.

Foods to limit

Some foods can trigger symptoms during a Crohn's flare. Examples include:
• whole grains
• fruits and vegetables with skins and seeds
• cruciferous vegetables, such as broccoli and cauliflower
• high fat foods, such as french fries, heavy cream, and bacon
• spicy foods
• caffeine, including in coffee and tea
• alcohol
• carbonated drinks, such as soda

However, keep in mind that trigger foods are different for each person. It may be helpful for a person to track their food and symptoms to see which foods trigger symptoms. A registered dietitian can also help a person determine which foods to avoid.

What to eat when in remission

When people are in remission from Crohn's disease, doctors typically recommend that they follow a nutritious, balanced diet that includes:
• whole grains, such as brown rice, quinoa, and others
• vegetables, including cruciferous vegetables
• fruit, including skin and seeds
These foods contain dietary fiber, which, in addition to bulking up stool, helps support the health of a person's gut microbiome. They can also reduce inflammation and support overall health.
People may have different fiber intake needs and foods to avoid, depending on their triggers. A doctor or dietitian can help determine a nutritious diet during remission from Crohn's disease.

Crohn's disease doesn't usually shorten your life. Most people with Crohn's disease are able to live productive and fulfilling lives, especially when they get effective treatment.

Is there a cure for Crohn's disease?

Existing treatments can't cure Crohn's disease, but they can help relieve symptoms, reduce flare-ups, and help you avoid possibly serious complications.

What to expect with Crohn's disease

Crohn's disease is a lifelong disease whose course varies a lot from person to person. Doctors can't predict how it will affect you. It might be mild or serious. You could have periods of symptoms that can last days, weeks, or months, followed by periods of remission that can last days, weeks, or years. There's often no way to predict when you'll have a flare.

Conditions Similar to Crohn's Disease

Ulcerative coitis, the other form of IBD, has symptoms very similar to those of Crohn's disease. It also tends to affect people younger than age 30. UC causes inflammation only in the colon, while Crohn's disease can affect any part of your digestive tract from the mouth to the anus. Crohn's disease usually affects your bowel in patches, but with UC, you have continuous stretches of inflammation.

Other conditions that could look like Crohn's disease include:

• Irritable bowel syndrome , a common digestive disorder whose symptoms may include abdominal pain, diarrhea, constipation, gas, or bloating.

• Celiac disease, an immune system reaction to gluten (a protein found in wheat, barley, and rye) that can damage your intestines. Symptoms include diarrhea, tiredness, and weight loss.

• Food allergy, in which certain foods trigger an allergic reaction in your body. Symptoms can include abdominal pain, diarrhea, and nausea. Some people have much more serious symptoms such as trouble breathing.

• Colon cancer, which could cause weight loss, abdominal pain, and blood in your poop.

One Pan Garlic Herb Chicken & Potatoes

Ingredients
1. 4 tablespoons olive oil
2. 1 tablespoon garlic
3. 1 teaspoon fresh rosemary
4. 1 teaspoon fresh thyme
5. 600 grams fresh skinless chicken breast
6. 4 potatoes, peeled and cut into chunks
7. ½ teaspoon salt
8. ½ teaspoon pepper
9. Olive oil for greasing the baking sheet

Instructions
1. Preheat oven to 400°F/200°C. Lightly grease a baking tray with olive oil.
2. Finely chop the garlic and herbs and add to a small bowl. Stir in the olive oil.
3. Arrange the chicken and potatoes on the prepared baking sheet. Pour half of the garlic herb mixture over top. Season with salt and pepper. Bake for 15 minutes.
4. Remove pan from oven. Flip chicken and stir potatoes. Drizzle with remaining garlic herb oil.
5. Bake for an additional 10-15 minutes, until chicken is cooked through and potatoes are crisp and golden.

Stir-Fried Chicken and Noodles

Ingredients
1. 2 tablespoons canola oil, divided
2. 600-800 grams fresh skinless chicken breast, cut into thin strips
3. 3 carrots, peeled and cut into thin 2-inch strips
4. 1 onion, quartered and thinly sliced
5. 2 garlic cloves, minced
6. ⅛ teaspoon salt1 teaspoon paprika
7. ½ teaspoon turmeric
8. ½ teaspoon sugar
9. 2 cups cooked thin rice noodles

Instructions
1. Heat 1 tablespoon of oil in a frying pan over medium heat. Add chicken and cook, stirring often, until browned. Add carrots, onion and garlic and cook, stirring often, until vegetables are tender.
2. In a small bowl, stir together the salt, paprika, turmeric, and sugar. Add the spice mixture to the pan and stir until the chicken and vegetables are evenly covered.
3. Add the cooked rice noodles and remaining 1 tablespoon of oil to the pan. Cook, stirring often, until the noodles are warm. Serve immediately.

2 Ingredient Banana Pancakes

Ingredients
1. 2 bananas
2. 2 eggs

3. Canola oil for greasing the pan

Instructions
1. Peel bananas and place in a medium bowl. Mash well with a fork.
2. Add the eggs to the bowl and stir until you have a custard- like consistency. The batter will be runny and have some small chunks of banana.
3. Heat a griddle or large skillet over medium heat. Lightly coat with canola oil.
4. When the pan is hot, spoon on 2 tablespoons of batter for each pancake. Cook for 1 minute, until the bottoms are browned and golden when lifted. Gently flip and cook for another minute on the other side.

Veggie Hash Browns

Ingredients
1. 3 potatoes, peeled and grated
2. ½ cup chopped fresh spinach
3. ½ white onion, finely chopped
4. ½ carrot, peeled and grated
5. ½ teaspoon salt
6. 1½ tablespoons white rice flour
7. 2 tablespoons canola oil

Instructions
1. Combine the potatoes, spinach, onion and carrot in a large bowl. Season with salt and mix well to combine.
2. Place the mixture in a clean kitchen towel and squeeze to remove any excess moisture. Return the veggie mix to the bowl and stir in the white rice flour.

3. Form the mixture into patties.
4. Heat the oil in a large pan over medium high heat. Gently drop in the hash brown patties. Cook for a few minutes on each side to brown. Lower the heat to medium and cook for several minutes more, until cooked through.

Banana Honey Muffins

Ingredients
1. 1 cup white rice flour
2. ½ teaspoon salt
3. 2 tablespoons sugar or honey
4. 1 egg
5. ¼ cup water
6. 2 tablespoons canola oil
7. 2 bananas, mashed
8. Canola oil for greasing muffin pan

Instructions
1. Preheat oven to 350°F/175°C and grease a 12 cup muffin pan with canola oil.
2. In a medium bowl stir together the rice flour, salt, and sugar (if using). In a small bowl, whisk the egg, water, canola oil, banana, and honey (if using). Add the wet ingredients to the dry ingredients and stir until well combined.
3. Spoon the batter evenly across 10 slots in the muffin pan. Bake for 15 minutes or until a toothpick inserted in the center of a muffin comes out clean.
4. Let muffins cool before removing from the pan.

Baked Chicken Nuggets

Ingredients
1. 1-2 teaspoons canola oil
2. 1-1½ cups white rice flour
3. 1 teaspoon cumin
4. 2 teaspoons paprika
5. ¼ teaspoon salt
6. ½ teaspoon pepper
7. 2 eggs
8. 1 kilogram fresh skinless chicken breast, cut into cubes
9. Canola oil for greasing baking dish

Instructions
1. Preheat oven to 350°F/175°C. Line two 23 x 33-centimeter baking sheets with aluminum foil and grease with canola oil.
2. In a small bowl combine the rice flour, cumin, paprika, salt, and pepper. In another small bowl, beat the eggs.
3. Using a pair of tongs, roll a piece of chicken in the flour mixture until covered on all sides. Dip the chicken into the eggs, roll in flour again, then place on a baking sheet. Repeat with remaining chicken.
4. Bake for 25-30 minutes, turning halfway through. The chicken should reach an internal temperature of 165°F/75°C.

Chicken Apple Potato Bake

Ingredients
1. 4 potatoes, peeled and quartered

2. 4 sweet apples, peeled, cored, and quartered
3. 4 tablespoons olive oil, divided
4. Salt and pepper
5. 600-800 grams fresh skinless chicken breast
6. 1 tablespoon chopped fresh thyme
7. ¼ cup chopped fresh parsley

Instructions
1. Bring 4 cups of water to a boil in a large saucepan. Add potatoes and apples. Reduce heat to a simmer and cook, covered, until tender, about 20 minutes.
2. Drain and transfer potatoes and apples to a large bowl. Toss with 2 tablespoons olive oil, salt and pepper.
3. Preheat oven to 177°C. Grease a large baking dish with olive oil and add potatoes and apples.
4. Sprinkle chicken with salt, pepper, thyme, and parsley; drizzle with remaining olive oil.
5. Add the chicken to baking dish and bake until cooked through, about 30 minutes.

Super Green Smoothie

Ingredients
1. 1 banana, frozen from fresh
2. ¼ avocado, peeled and pit removed
3. ½ cup fresh spinach leaves
4. 250 mL prepared Modulen

Instructions
1. Add all ingredients to a blender and blend until smooth. Store bought frozen foods are not allowed on the Crohn's

Disease Exclusion diet. Freeze your own fresh fruit to use in smoothies.

Chicken Pita

Ingredients
1. 1 serving Pita Bread
2. 1 serving Baked Chicken Breast
3. ½ tomato, chopped
4. 1 lettuce leaf, chopped or shredded
5. 1 teaspoon fresh parsley
6. Fresh lemon wedge

Instructions
1. Layer the chicken, tomato and lettuce on top of the pita bread.
2. Top with parsley and a squeeze of fresh lemon juice.

Lemon & Garlic Chicken

Ingredients
1. 600-800 grams fresh skinless chicken breast
2. ¼ cup fresh lemon juice
3. 2 tablespoons olive oil
4. ½ teaspoon sea salt
5. ½ teaspoon pepper
6. 3 garlic cloves
7. ½ cup fresh parsley, chopped

Instructions

1. Whisk together the lemon juice, olive oil, salt and pepper in a large bowl. Stir in the garlic and parsley. Add the chicken to the marinade and turn to coat. Let marinate in the refrigerator for up to 2 hours.
2. Preheat oven to 400°F/200°C.
3. Transfer chicken and marinade to a baking dish. Cover loosely with parchment paper. Bake for about 30-40 minutes, until the chicken reaches an internal temperature of 165°F/75°C.
4. Serve chicken drizzled with the lemon oil mixture from the baking dish.

Rice Pudding

Ingredients
1. ½ cup dry white rice
2. 1½ cups water
3. 2 teaspoons sugar
4. ½ teaspoon cinnamon
5. 1 banana, mashed

Instructions
1. Stir together the rice, water, sugar, and cinnamon in a small pot. Bring to a gentle boil over medium-high heat. Reduce heat to low and cook for 13 minutes, stirring occasionally.
2. Remove pan from heat. Stir in banana. Add more water if the pudding is too thick.
3. Serve warm.

Scrambled Eggs

Ingredients
1. 1 teaspoon canola oil
2. 2 eggs
3. Salt and pepper

Instructions
1. Heat oil in a large nonstick pan over medium heat.
2. Whisk together the eggs, salt, and pepper in a medium bowl. Add egg mixture to the hot pan.
3. As the eggs start to set, gently pull mixture across the pan, forming soft curds. Continue to let eggs cook, occasionally folding the mixture until it has thickened and no liquid remains.
4. Remove from heat and serve immediately.

Quick Orange Squares

Ingredients
1. 4 eggs
2. 1 cup sugar
3. 1 cup freshly squeezed orange juice
4. 2 cups white rice flour
5. 3/4 cup canola oil
6. Canola oil for greasing baking dish

Instructions
1. Preheat the oven to 350°F/175°C. Grease a 20 x 20-centimeter baking dish with canola oil.

2. Whisk together all the ingredients in a large bowl. Pour the batter into the prepared baking dish and spread out evenly.
3. Bake for 30 minutes or until a toothpick inserted in the center comes out clean.
4. Let cool before cutting into 12 pieces.

Baked Potato Chips

Ingredients
1. 2 potatoes, peeled and very thinly sliced (using a knife or a mandolin)
2. Salt and pepper
3. Optional seasonings: paprika, cumin

Instructions
1. Place potato slices in a bowl of water. Let soak for 30 minutes to remove excess starch.
2. Preheat oven to 400°F/200°C. Line a large baking sheet with parchment paper.
3. Transfer potatoes to a paper towel and pat dry. Add salt, pepper, and additional seasonings if desired. Arrange the potato slices on the prepared baking sheet in a single layer.
4. Bake for about 10 minutes, until browned and crispy.

Mediterranean Mashed Potatoes

Ingredients
1. 4 potatoes, peeled and cut into chunks

2. 1 teaspoon coarse salt
3. ¼ cup olive oil
4. 1 teaspoon finely chopped fresh basil
5. 1 teaspoon finely chopped fresh parsley
6. 1 teaspoon finely chopped fresh tarragon
7. Salt and pepper

Instructions
1. Place potatoes in a large saucepan and cover with cold water. Stir in the salt. Bring to a boil over high heat.
2. Reduce heat to a simmer and cook for about 10 minutes, until the potatoes are fork-tender.
3. Set aside ½ cup of the cooking liquid; drain off the rest. Transfer the potatoes to a bowl.
4. Add oil and reserved cooking liquid to the saucepan; let warm for several minutes over medium heat.
5. In the meantime, mash the potatoes, either by hand or using a ricer or food mill. Add the mashed potatoes back to the saucepan.
6. Stir in the basil, parsley, and tarragon. Season with salt and pepper.

Bruschetta Chicken

Ingredients
1. 150-200 grams fresh skinless chicken breast
2. ½ cup chopped tomato
3. 1 tablespoon olive oil
4. Squeeze of fresh lemon juice
5. 5 fresh basil leaves, chopped
6. Salt and pepper
7. 1 cup fresh spinach leaves

Instructions
1. Preheat oven to 375°F/190°C.
2. Season chicken with salt and pepper on each side. Bake for about 35-40 minutes, until cooked through.
3. In the meantime, mix together the chopped tomatoes, oil, lemon juice, basil, and a sprinkle of salt and pepper. Do this as soon as the chicken goes in the oven, so that the flavors have time to blend together.
4. Serve the cooked chicken with the fresh spinach and the tomato mixture.

Pancakes

Ingredients
1. 1 cup white rice flour
2. 3 tablespoons honey
3. 1 egg, beaten
4. ¾ cup water, divided
5. 2 tablespoons canola oil
6. ¼ teaspoon salt
7. Canola oil for greasing the frying pan

Instructions
1. In large bowl, stir together all the ingredients.
2. Heat a small amount of canola oil in a frying pan over medium heat. Pour 1/4 cup of batter onto the pan. Cook until the top of the pancake starts to bubble and the bottom is golden, about 2 minutes. Flip the pancake and continue cooking until the other side is golden, about 1-2 minutes.
3. Repeat until all the batter has been used.

Banana Smoothie

Ingredients
1. 250 mL prepared Modulen®
2. 2 bananas
3. 2 teaspoons honey
4. Pinch of ground cinnamon
5. Seeds from ¼ vanilla bean

Instructions
1. Combine all ingredients in a blender and blend until smooth.

Chicken Bolognese

Ingredients
1. ⅓ cup packed fresh basil leaves, roughly chopped
2. 2 tablespoons olive oil
3. 600-800 grams fresh skinless chicken breast, freshly ground
4. 1 medium onion, diced
5. 2 carrots, peeled and diced
6. 5 tomatoes, chopped
7. 3 cloves garlic, minced
8. 1 cup water½ teaspoon pepper
9. ¼ teaspoon salt

Instructions
1. Heat oil in a frying pan over medium-high heat. Add the ground chicken to the pan and cook, stirring often, until no

longer pink. Add the onion, carrots, and garlic and cook, stirring often, until the onion is soft.

2. Add the tomatoes and water to the pan and increase heat to high. When the sauce is boiling, reduce heat to low and simmer for 1 hour.

3. When the sauce is finished cooking, stir in the basil, pepper, and salt.

Crunchy Cookies

Ingredients
1. ½ cup canola oil
2. ½ cup sugar
3. 2 egg whites
4. 1¼ cup white rice flour
5. Zest of ½ lemon

Instructions
1. Preheat oven to 350°F/175°C and line two 23 x 33-centimeter baking sheets with parchment paper.

2. Combine all the ingredients in a large bowl. Form the dough into a large ball.

3. Put a large piece of parchment paper on the counter. Put the dough in the middle of the paper and put another piece of parchment paper on top. Using a rolling pin, roll out the dough between the parchment paper until it is 1⁄2 centimeter thick.

4. Using a medium cookie cutter of your choice, cut the dough into 18 cookies, re-rolling the dough as needed. Arrange the cookies on the prepared baking sheets.

5. Bake for 10 minutes. Let cookies cool before removing from the baking sheets.

Chicken Burger

Ingredients
1. 450 grams fresh skinless chicken breast, freshly ground
2. 1 small carrot, peeled and grated
3. 2 green onions, minced
4. 1 teaspoon salt
5. 1 teaspoon pepper
6. 2 tablespoons chopped fresh parsley
7. 2 tablespoons chopped fresh basil
8. Canola oil

Instructions
1. Heat a large nonstick or iron skillet over medium heat. Lightly coat the pan with canola oil.
2. Combine the chicken, vegetables, and seasonings in a large bowl. Gently mix together with your hands. Form into 3 patties.
3. Place the patties in the hot pan and cook for about 15 minutes, turning once about halfway through the cooking time. The chicken is cooked through when it reaches an internal temperature of 165°F/75°C.

Orange Juice Cake

Ingredients
1. 5 egg whites
2. ¼ teaspoon salt
3. 1 cup sugar, divided
4. 3 egg yolks
5. ½ cup canola oil

6. Zest of 1 small lemon
7. 2 cups white rice flour
8. 1 cup freshly squeezed orange juice
9. Canola oil for greasing the baking dish

Instructions
1. Preheat oven to 350°F/175°C and grease a 20 x 20-centimeter baking dish with canola oil.
2. Using a handheld mixer, beat the egg whites, salt, and 1/2 cup of sugar together in a medium bowl until soft peaks form.
3. In a separate bowl, whisk together the egg yolks and remaining 1/2 cup of sugar. Add the oil and lemon zest and whisk. Slowly fold in the rice flour and orange juice, alternating between the two (starting and ending with the rice flour). Fold in the egg whites.
4. Pour the batter into the prepared baking dish and spread out evenly.
5. Bake for 45 minutes or until a toothpick inserted in the center comes out clean. Let cake cool before cutting into 12 pieces.

Baked Chicken & Potatoes

Ingredients
1. 4 potatoes, peeled and cut into cubes
2. 3 tablespoons olive oil, divided
3. ¾ teaspoon salt
4. ½ teaspoon pepper
5. 4 cloves garlic, minced
6. 1 lemon - ½ juiced, ½ cut into wedges
7. 4 fresh skinless chicken breasts (about 700-800 grams)

8. 2 tablespoons chopped fresh cilantro or parsley

Instructions
1. Preheat oven to 218°C.
2. Place potatoes in a large baking dish. Toss with 1 tablespoon oil, salt and pepper. Bake for about 30 minutes.
3. Heat the remaining 2 tablespoons of oil in a small skillet over medium heat. Add garlic and cook, stirring frequently, for about 2 minutes, until lightly golden. Remove pan from heat. Stir in lemon juice.
4. Remove baking dish from oven. Push the potatoes to the sides. Place chicken in the middle; drizzle with the lemon garlic mixture. Bake for about 20 minutes, until chicken is cooked through and potatoes are tender.
5. Transfer chicken to a plate. Add cilantro or parsley to the baking dish and mix with the potatoes.
6. Serve the chicken and potatoes with lemon wedges.

Breakfast Potatoes

Ingredients
1. 4 potatoes, peeled and cut into cubes
2. 2 tablespoons canola oil
3. 1 teaspoon salt
4. ¼ teaspoon pepper

Instructions
1. Preheat the oven to 400°F/200°C. Line a large baking sheet with foil or parchment paper.
2. Place potatoes in a large bowl. Drizzle with oil and toss to coat. Add salt and pepper and toss again.

3. Arrange the potatoes in an even layer on the prepared baking sheet.
4. Bake for 20-25 minutes. Remove potatoes from oven and stir.
5. Return pan to oven and broil for about 5 minutes, until potatoes are browned and crisp.

Spinach & Tomato Scramble

Ingredients
1. 2 eggs
2. ½ medium tomato, chopped
3. ½ cup fresh spinach leaves
4. Pinch of salt and pepper
5. 1 teaspoon canola oil

Instructions
1. Heat oil in a medium nonstick skillet over medium heat.
2. Add tomatoes and spinach to the pan. Season with salt and pepper. Cook for several minutes, until the spinach has wilted.
3. Crack the eggs into a small bowl and whisk well to combine. Pour the eggs into the pan over the cooked vegetables. Use a spatula to move the eggs around the pan until they are set.
4. Serve immediately.

Sautéed Chicken & Apples

Ingredients
1. 1 tablespoon olive oil
2. 1 small sweet onion, thinly sliced
3. 2 red apples, peeled and sliced
4. 400 grams fresh skinless chicken breast, sliced into strips
5. ½ teaspoon salt
6. ¼ teaspoon pepper
7. 1-2 teaspoons fresh rosemary, finely chopped
8. 1 tablespoon fresh lemon juice

Instructions
1. Heat oil in a large sauté pan over medium-high heat.
2. Add onion and apple slices to the pan. Cook for about 5 minutes, until browned and softened.
3. In the meantime, place chicken in a small bowl and toss with salt, pepper and rosemary.
4. Push the onions and apples to the sides of the pan. Place chicken in the center. Cook for about 6-8 minutes, turning occasionally, until the chicken is browned on both sides.
5. Add lemon juice to the pan. Cover, turn heat down to medium, and cook 3-5 minutes more, until the chicken is cooked through.

Parmesan-Crusted Chicken

Ingredients
1. 100g (3½ oz) day-old white breadcrumbs
2. 50g (1¾ oz) finely grated Parmesan cheese
3. 2 garlic cloves, crushed

4. handful of basil leaves
5. finely grated zest of 1 lemon
6. salt and freshly ground black pepper1 large egg, beaten
7. 1 heaped tbsp plain flour
8. 8 skin-on bone-in chicken thighs
9. 2 tbsp olive oil

Instructions
1. Preheat the oven to 200°C (400°F/Gas 6). In a food processor, place the breadcrumbs, Parmesan, garlic, basil, zest, and salt and pepper, and process until the basil turns the mixture green. Tip into a wide, shallow bowl.
2. Place the egg in a shallow bowl and the flour in a freezer bag. Season the flour well. Put the chicken in the freezer bag and toss to coat. Tip out into a sieve and shake to remove excess flour.
3. Dip each piece of chicken in the egg, then coat well in the breadcrumbs.
4. Heat the olive oil on a large baking tray for 5 minutes, then arrange the chicken on the tray, spaced well apart and in a single layer. Cook for 40–45 minutes, turning occasionally, until golden brown and crispy.

Avocado Deviled Eggs

Ingredients
1. 6 hard boiled eggs
2. 1 medium avocado
3. 2 teaspoons fresh lemon juice
4. Pinch of salt and pepper

Instructions

1. Peel the hard boiled eggs and cut in half lengthwise. Scoop out the yolks and transfer to a medium bowl.
2. Cut the avocado in half and remove the pit. Scoop the flesh into the bowl with the egg yolks.
3. Add the lemon juice, salt and pepper to the bowl. Use a fork to mash all of the ingredients together until combined.
4. Fill each of the egg halves with some of the avocado mixture.

Potato Salad

Ingredients
1. 2 potatoes, peeled and cut into cubes
2. 3 eggs½ onion, minced
3. 2 tablespoons olive oil
4. 3 tablespoons fresh lemon juice
5. Salt and pepper
Instructions
1. Put the potatoes in a small pot and cover with water. Bring to a boil over high heat, then reduce heat to medium-low. Cook the potatoes until tender but still slightly firm, about 8-10 minutes.
2. In the meantime, put the eggs in another small pot and cover with water. Bring to a boil over high heat, then reduce heat to low and cook for 10 minutes. Rinse eggs with cold water and set aside to cool for 5-10 minutes. When the eggs are cool, remove the shells, then chop.
3. In a medium bowl, combine the potatoes, eggs, onion, olive oil, lemon juice, and some salt and pepper. Stir well to combine.

Potato Rosti

Ingredients
1. 400g (14oz) waxy potatoes, such as Charlottes, peeledsalt and freshly ground black pepper
2. 1 tbsp butter
3. 1 tbsp olive oil

Instructions
1. Bring the whole, peeled potatoes to the boil in a large pan of salted water. Reduce to a simmer and cook for 7–10 minutes, depending on size, until part-cooked but still firm. Leave to cool, then grate coarsely and toss with salt and pepper.
2. Melt the butter and oil in a 20–22cm (8–8 ½ in) frying pan. Put the potato in the pan and squash it down with a spatula to make a large, flat pancake. Cook over a medium heat for 5–7 minutes, until crispy underneath.
3. To turn, slide the potato pancake onto a large plate. Put another plate on top and flip the whole thing over, so the cooked side is uppermost. Slide back into the pan and cook for a further 5–7 minutes until crispy underneath. Cut into wedges to serve.

Strawberry Banana Smoothie

Ingredients
1. 500mL prepared Modulen®
2. 1 banana, fresh or frozen*
3. 3 strawberries, fresh or frozen*

Instructions
1. Place all of the ingredients in a blender and blend until smooth.

Sugar-Spiced Chicken

Ingredients
1. 600 grams fresh skinless chicken breast
2. ¼ cup sugar
3. 2 tablespoons paprika
4. 1 tablespoon fresh oregano
5. 3 tablespoons minced garlic
6. ¼ teaspoon salt
7. ½ teaspoon pepper

Instructions
1. Combine the sugar and spices in a large bowl. Add the chicken to bowl and toss to coat evenly with the seasoning mixture. Cover and refrigerate for 1-3 hours.
2. Preheat oven to 425°F/220°C.
3. Arrange the chicken on a lined baking sheet and bake for 20-25 minutes, until chicken is golden brown and cooked through.

Baked Bananas

Ingredients
1. Canola oil
2. 4 bananas, peeled and halved lengthwise
3. 4 teaspoons honey

4. 1 tablespoon ground cinnamon
5. 1-inch piece fresh ginger, peeled and grated

Instructions
1. Preheat the oven to 375°F/190°C. Lightly grease a baking dish with canola oil.
2. Place the banana halves on the prepared baking dish. Drizzle with honey, then top with cinnamon and ginger.
3. Cover with foil and bake for 10-15 minutes, until heated through.

Carrot Fries

Ingredients
1. 10 medium carrots, peeled, ends trimmed
2. 2 tablespoons olive oil
3. Salt and pepper

Instructions
1. Preheat oven to 218°C. Line a baking sheet with aluminum foil.
2. Cut each carrot in half crosswise. Then cut each half in half lengthwise, and the resulting halves lengthwise again. This will give you 8 sticks from each carrot.
3. Coat the sliced carrots with oil and season with salt and pepper.
4. Arrange the carrots on the prepared baking sheet in a single layer.
5. Bake for about 20 minutes, until the carrots are tender.

Rice Flour Crepes

Ingredients
1. 3 tablespoons sugar
2. 3 eggs
3. ¾ cup white rice flour
4. ½ cup water
5. 2 tablespoons canola oil
6. ⅛ teaspoon salt
7. Canola oil for greasing the frying pan
8. Suggested fillings: sliced banana, sliced strawberries, peeled sliced apple, cinnamon, sugar, honey

Instructions
1. In a medium bowl, stir together all the ingredients. Let the batter sit for 15 minutes.
2. Heat a small amount of canola oil in a frying pan over medium-high heat. Stir the batter until it is smooth again. Pour ⅓ cup of the batter onto the pan. Tilt the pan quickly to spread the batter over the whole pan. Flip the crepe after 30 seconds and cook for another 30 seconds on the other side. Remove from the pan and put on a plate. Repeat until all the batter has been used, adding more canola oil to the pan between crepes.
3. Fill the crepes with desired fillings and roll or fold up.

Fresh Herb Pesto

Ingredients
1. ½ cup tightly packed fresh cilantro leaves
2. ½ cup tightly packed fresh parsley leaves

3. ½ cup tightly packed fresh basil leaves
4. ½ cup olive oil

Instructions
1. Put all the ingredients in the bowl of a food processor.
Process until the mixture is smooth.

Chicken Spread

Ingredients
1. 1 teaspoon + 3 tablespoons canola oil
2. ½ onion, chopped
3. 1 small fresh skinless chicken breast (about 5 ounces),
cut into cubes

Instructions
1. Heat 1 teaspoon of canola oil in a frying pan over
medium- high heat. Add chicken and cook, stirring often,
until it is no longer pink. Add the onion and continue
cooking until the onion is soft.
2. Remove from heat and let cool for 5 minutes.
3. Put the chicken and onion in the bowl of a food
processor. Add 3 tablespoons of canola oil. Process until
smooth. For Phase 1, serve on a Savory Cream Puff or with
Rosemary Garlic Rice Crackers. In Phase 2 and 3, spread
may be served on homemade bread.

Baked Avocado Eggs

Ingredients
1. 1 avocado2 eggsSalt and pepper

Instructions
1. Preheat oven to 425°F/220°C.
2. Slice the avocado in half lengthwise and remove the pit. Scoop out a few spoon fulls from the center of the avocado to create a larger cavity. Place the avocado halves skin side down in a baking dish.
3. Gently crack one egg into each half. Season with salt and pepper.
4. Bake for about 15-20 minutes, until the eggs are set.

Mayonnaise

Ingredients
1. 2 egg yolks
2. 2 tablespoons water
3. 2 tablespoons fresh lemon juice
4. 1 teaspoon sugar
5. ½ teaspoon salt
6. 1 cup canola oil

Instructions
1. Fill a large bowl 3⁄4 full with ice water and set aside.
2. Put 5-8 centimeters of water in a small saucepan and bring to a boil over medium-high heat.
3. Whisk together the egg yolks, water, lemon juice, sugar, and salt in a small bowl that will fit tightly on the saucepan.

When the water is boiling, reduce heat to medium-low. Put the bowl on top of the saucepan (the water in the saucepan should not touch the bottom of the bowl). Whisk the yolk mixture constantly, until it reaches 72°C. Increase heat as needed to keep the water at a gentle boil.
4. Put the small bowl in the ice water. Whisk the yolk mixture until it is room temperature. Remove bowl from water.
5. Pour about 1 tablespoon of canola oil into the yolk mixture and whisk until well combined. Repeat until all of the oil has been added to the yolk mixture.
6. Store in an airtight container in the refrigerator for up 4 days.

Tuscan Chicken With Sage

Ingredients
1. 3 tablespoons olive oil
2. 30 fresh sage leaves
3. 1-2 garlic cloves, thinly sliced
4. 4 fresh skinless chicken breasts (600-800 grams), butterflied
5. Coarse salt to taste

Instructions
1. Pour the olive oil into a frying pan and spread evenly over pan. Arrange the sage leaves and garlic on top of the oil. Heat the frying pan over medium-high heat.
2. When the pan is hot, add the chicken. Turn the chicken breasts over when the meat is white. Sprinkle with salt and continue cooking until the chicken reaches an internal temperature of 165°F/75°C.

Potato Pizza Margherita

Ingredients
1. 2 lb baking potatoes, peeled and cut into small chunks
2. 3 tablespoons olive oil, plus extra for oiling
3. 1 egg, beaten
4. ½ cup Parmesan or cheddar cheese, grated
5. 4 tablespoons sundried tomato paste or tomato ketchup
6. 1 lb small tomatoes, thinly sliced
7. 4 oz mozzarella cheese, thinly sliced
8. 1 tablespoon chopped thyme, plus extra sprigs to garnish (optional)
9. salt

Instructions
1. Cook the potatoes in a saucepan of salted boiling water for 15 minutes or until tender. Drain well, return to the pan, and let cool for 10 minutes.
2. Add 2 tablespoons of the oil, the egg, and half the grated Parmesan to the potato and mix well. Turn out onto an oiled baking sheet and spread out to form a 10 inch round. Place in a preheated oven, 400°F, for 15 minutes.
3. Remove from the oven and spread with the tomato paste or ketchup. Arrange the tomato and mozzarella slices on top. Sprinkle with the remaining grated Parmesan, thyme, if using, and a little salt. Drizzle with the remaining oil.
4. Return to the oven for an additional 15 minutes until the potato is crisp around the edges and the cheese is melting. Cut into generous wedges, garnish with thyme sprigs, if liked, and serve.

Strawberry Banana Sorbet

Ingredients
1. 2 bananas, sliced
2. 4 medium strawberries, sliced
3. 1 tablespoon sugar
4. ¼ cup fresh squeezed orange juice (yield from ½ large orange)

Instructions
1. Put the sliced fruit in an airtight container and freeze for 24 hours.
2. Thaw the fruit at room temperature for 10 minutes. Put the fruit in the bowl of a food processor and add the sugar and orange juice. Process until the mixture is smooth and looks like ice cream. If needed, scrape down the bowl during processing.
3. Put the sorbet in an airtight container and freeze for 20-30 minutes before serving. If freezing for longer, thaw at room temperature for 5-10 minutes before serving.

Crispy Risotto Cakes

Ingredients
1. 800g (1¾ lb) cooked, cold risotto, such as Simple Parmesan risotto
2. 50g (1¾ oz) finely grated Parmesan cheese
3. handful of flat-leaf parsley or basil leaves, finely chopped (optional)
4. salt and freshly ground black pepperolive oil, for brushing

Instructions
1. Preheat the oven to 230°C (450°F/Gas 8). In a bowl, mix together the risotto, Parmesan, and herbs (if using), and season well.
2. Use a 10cm (4in) round cutter or mould to make cakes of the mixture: place the cutter or mould on a work surface and spoon in one-quarter of the risotto mixture, squashing it in and flattening it off nicely. Remove the cutter or mould. Repeat to make 4 cakes.
3. Brush each risotto cake with a little oil on one side and place oil-side down on a non-stick baking tray. Brush the upper side with oil and bake at the top of the oven for 25 minutes, turning carefully after 15 minutes, or until golden and crispy on the outside but soft and yielding within.

Sweet Cream Puffs

Ingredients
1. 1½ cups water
2. ½ cup canola oil
3. 2 teaspoons sugar
4. 1 cup white rice flour
5. 4 eggs

Instructions
1. Preheat oven to 420°F/215°C. Line two 23 x 33-centimeter baking sheets with parchment paper.
2. Stir together the water, canola oil, and sugar in a medium pot and bring to a gentle boil over high heat.
3. Remove pan from heat. Add the rice flour and stir quickly until combined. Let cool for 5 minutes.

4. Using an upright mixer with a kneading hook or a handheld mixer, add 1 egg to the dough and combine. Repeat with remaining eggs.
5. Drop the dough by 1/4 cup onto the prepared baking sheets, 2 inches apart. Bake for 10 minutes.
6. Lower the oven temperature to 400°F/200°C and bake for another 25 minutes.
7. Remove puffs from the oven. Transfer to a cooling rack after 5 minutes.
8. Store at room temperature for up to 24 hours, or freeze.

Chicken Orzo Salad

Ingredients
1. 11oz peeled cucumber chopped
2. 2 cups orzo pasta
3. ½ cup chopped green onions (scallions)
4. 1 cup frozen peas, thawed
5. ⅓ cup water
6. ½ cup crumbled reduced-fat feta cheese
7. 2 teaspoons dried dill weed leaves
8. 3 tablespoons lemon juice
9. 8 ounces sun-dried tomatoes, sliced, reconstituted, and drained
10. 1 teaspoon minced garlic
11. 2 cups skinless, cooked chicken breast
12. 2 tablespoons olive oil.
13. 15 tsp salt

Instructions
1. Cook orzo according to package directions. Drain.

2. In large bowl, combine orzo, chicken, peas, green onions, feta, cucumber, toma-toes, dill.
3. In another bowl, whisk together reserved sun dried tomato water with remaining ingredients.
4. Toss with orzo mixture. Refrigerate for at least 1 hour before serving.

Breakfast Berry Bars

Ingredients
1. oil, for greasing
2. 397g can sweetened condensed milk
3. 300g (10oz) mixed dried berries, such as cranberries, blueberries, and sour cherries
4. 250g (9oz) rolled oats50g (1¾oz) crispy rice
5. 30g (1oz) sunflower seeds
6. 30g (1oz) pumpkin seeds

Instructions
1. Preheat the oven to 160°C (325°F/Gas 3). Lightly oil the baking tray.
2. Gently heat the condensed milk in a large, heavy pan and slowly bring to the boil. Remove it from the heat, then tip in the fruit, oats, crispy rice, and seeds. Mix well with a wooden spoon.
3. Tip into the prepared tin, then level the surface with the back of a wetted spoon. Bake for 30–35 minutes or until pale golden.
4. Remove from the oven, cool in the tin for 5 minutes, and cut into 16 bars. Transfer the bars to a wire rack to cool completely. Store in an airtight container for up to 1 week.

Summer Salad

Ingredients
1. 4 tomatoes, cut into wedges
2. 1 cucumber, peeled and sliced into half moons
3. 1 avocado, pitted, peeled and cubed
4. ¼ red onion, thinly sliced
5. ¼ cup chopped fresh basil
6. 2 tablespoons olive oil
7. Juice of one lemon
8. Salt and pepper

Instructions
1. Combine the tomatoes, cucumber, avocado, red onion and basil in a large bowl.
2. Drizzle with oil and squeeze fresh lemon juice over top. Season with salt and pepper. Toss gently to combine.

Baked Salmon With Cucumber Dill Sauce

Ingredients
1. ½ cucumbersalt and freshly ground black pepper
2. 250g (9oz) plain yogurt
3. 2 tsp Dijon mustard
4. 1 spring onion, finely chopped
5. 1 tbsp chopped dill
6. 4 salmon steaks or fillets, skinned
7. 2 tsp olive oil
8. juice of ½ lemon

Instructions

1. Finely dice the cucumber and place in a sieve over a bowl. Sprinkle with salt and leave to drain for 1 hour. Rinse with cold water and pat dry with kitchen paper. Stir the drained cucumber into the yogurt and add the mustard, spring onion, and dill. Season to taste with salt and pepper. Set aside.

2. Preheat the oven to 200°C (400°F/Gas 6). Arrange the salmon fillets in a shallow baking dish, brush with oil, and season to taste with salt and pepper.

3. Sprinkle the salmon with lemon juice and roast for 8–10 minutes, depending on the thickness, until just cooked through but still moist inside. Remove from the oven and stir the juices from the dish into the cucumber sauce.

4. Serve the salmon hot or cold, with the sauce spooned over it.

Apple & Banana Smoothie

Ingredients
1. 1 apple, peeled and chopped
2. 1 banana, frozen from fresh
3. 1 teaspoon honey
4. 250 mL prepared Modulen®

Instructions
1. Combine all ingredients in a blender and blend until smooth. Store bought frozen foods are not allowed on the Crohn's Disease Exclusion diet. Freeze your own fresh fruit to use in smoothies.

Fluffy Omelet Strips

Ingredients
1. 2 eggs
2. Salt and pepper
3. 1 tablespoon canola oil

Instructions
1. Heat oil in a small non-stick skillet over medium heat.
2. Crack the eggs into a medium bowl and whisk well, until frothy. Season with salt and pepper.
3. Add eggs to the pan. Cook for 2-3 minutes, using a rubber spatula to lift the edges and tilting the pan to let the uncooked eggs run underneath. Flip the omelet and cook for about 30 seconds more, until the eggs are set.
4. Remove pan from heat. Let omelet cool slightly before slicing into strips.

Chicken, Lemon & Olive Stew

Ingredients
1. 1.5 kg (3 lb) chickenabout 4 tablespoons olive oil
2. 12 baby onions, peeled but left whole
3. 2 garlic cloves, crushed
4. 1 teaspoon each ground cumin, ginger and turmeric
5. ½ teaspoon ground cinnamon
6. 450 ml (¾ pint) chicken stock (see page 16)
7. 125 g (4 oz) kalamata olives1 preserved lemon, pulp and skin discarded, chopped

8. 2 tablespoons chopped fresh coriandersalt and pepper

Instructions
1. Joint the chicken into 8 pieces (or ask your butcher to do this for you). Heat the oil in a flameproof casserole and brown the chicken on all sides. Remove the pieces with a slotted spoon and set aside.
2. Add the onions, garlic and spices and sauté over a low heat for 10 minutes until just golden. Return the chicken to the pan, stir in the stock and bring to the boil. Cover and simmer gently for 30 minutes.
3. Add the olives, preserved lemon and coriander and cook for a further 15 –20 minutes until the chicken is really tender. Taste and adjust the seasoning, if necessary.

Banana Pancakes

Ingredients
1. 2 very ripe bananas, mashed
2. 2 eggs
3. 2 tablespoons white rice flour
4. 1 tablespoon sugar
5. ½ teaspoon cinnamon
6. Canola oil for greasing the frying pan

Instructions
1. In a medium bowl stir together all the ingredients.
2. Heat a small amount of canola oil in a frying pan over medium heat. Pour 1/4 cup of batter into the pan and cook until the bottom of the pancake is browned or bubbles form on the top, about 2-3 minutes. Flip the pancake and

continue cooking until the other side is browned, about 2 minutes.

3. Repeat until all the batter has been used.

Fried Chicken Nuggets

Ingredients
1. 2½ cups white rice flour, divided
2. 1 teaspoon + 1 tablespoon paprika, divided
3. 1½ teaspoons cumin, divided
4. ½ teaspoon salt, divided
5. ½ teaspoon pepper, divided
6. 2 cups carbonated water
7. 900 grams fresh skinless chicken breast, cut into cubes
8. Canola oil for frying

Instructions
1. To make the seasoned rice flour, stir together 1/2 cup of rice flour, 1 teaspoon paprika, 1/2 teaspoon cumin, 1/4 teaspoon salt, and 1/4 teaspoon pepper in a small bowl.
2. To make the batter, stir together the remaining rice flour, paprika, cumin, salt, pepper, and the carbonated water in a medium bowl.
3. Heat a frying pan with 1/2 centimeter of canola oil in it over medium-high heat. Dip each piece of chicken in the seasoned rice flour, then in the batter, and put in the pan.
4. Cook chicken for 5 minutes, turning halfway through. The chicken should reach an internal temperature of 165°F/75°C.

Huevos Rancheros

Ingredients
1. 2 tablespoons olive oil
2. 1 large onion, diced
3. 2 red peppers, deseeded and diced
4. 2 garlic cloves, crushed
5. ¾ teaspoon dried oregano
6. 400 g (13 oz) can chopped tomatoes
7. 4 eggs
8. 20 g (¾ oz) feta cheese, crumbled
9. 4 toasted gluten-free pitta breads, to serve

Instructions
1. Heat the oil in a frying pan over a medium heat, then add the onion, peppers, garlic and oregano and cook for 5 minutes.
2. Add the tomatoes and cook for a further 5 minutes. Pour the tomato mixture into a shallow ovenproof dish and make 4 dips in the mixture.
3. Crack the eggs into the dips, sprinkle with the feta and cook under a preheated hot grill for 3–4 minutes.
4. Serve with toasted pitta breads.

Chicken, Bacon, Vegetable and Cheese Layers

Ingredients
1. 4 tablespoons olive oil
2. 2 chicken breasts, each about 150 g (5 oz), thinly sliced
3. 175 g (6 oz) streaky bacon, chopped
4. 375 g (12 oz) butternut squash, thinly sliced

5. 1 red onion, thinly sliced
6. 4 large tomatoes, sliced
7. 150 g (5 oz) mature Cheddar cheese, grated
8. 4 tablespoons chopped parsley (optional)

Instructions
1. Heat the oil in a large, heavy-based frying pan and cook the chicken breasts and bacon over a high heat for 3 minutes. Add the thinly sliced butternut squash and onion and continue cooking over a high heat for 10 minutes.
2. Put a layer of one-half of the sliced tomatoes in the base of a shallow, ovenproof dish. Spoon half the chicken and butternut mixture over the top. Scatter over one-half of the grated cheese. Top with a further layer of tomatoes and the remaining chicken and butternut and a layer of cheese.
3. Cook under a preheated moderate grill for 10–15 minutes or until golden and bubbling. Garnish with parsley, if liked, and serve with a simple crisp green salad.

Potato and Onion Omelet

Ingredients
1. 2 potatoes, peeled
2. ¼ cup chopped fresh parsley
3. 4 eggs, beaten
4. ½ onion, diced
5. Salt and pepper to taste
6. Canola oil for frying

Instructions

1. Grate the potatoes using a cheese grater. Squeeze the water out of the grated potatoes by pressing them between two dishcloths.
2. Put the potatoes in a medium bowl. Stir in the parsley, eggs, onion, salt, and pepper.
3. Heat a small amount of oil in a frying pan over medium heat. Pour in half the egg mixture and spread out evenly with the back of a spoon. Cook for about 4 minutes, until the edges begin to brown. Flip the omelet and cook for 4 minutes on the other side.
4. Remove the omelet from the pan and repeat with the remaining egg mixture.

Banana Orange Avocado Smoothie

Ingredients
1. 2 bananas, frozen from fresh
2. ¾ cup freshly squeezed orange juice (yield from about 2 large oranges)
3. 1 avocado

Instructions
1. Combine all ingredients in a blender and blend until smooth.

Hidden Vegetable Pasta Sauce

Ingredients
1. 2 tbsp olive oil
2. 1 onion, finely chopped

3. 1 small carrot, finely chopped
4. ½ celery stick, finely chopped
5. ¼ red pepper, finely chopped
6. ¼ yellow pepper, finely chopped
7. 5cm (2in) piece of courgette, finely chopped
8. 1 garlic clove, crushed
9. 400g can of chopped tomatoes
10. 1 tbsp tomato puréefreshly ground black pepper (optional)

Instructions
1. Heat the oil in a heavy-based saucepan and cook the onion, carrot, and celery over a medium heat for 5 minutes, until softened, but not browned. Add the peppers and courgette and cook for 2–3 minutes, then add the garlic and cook for a final minute.
2. Now add the tomatoes. Half- fill the empty can with water and add that too, with the tomato purée. Bring to the boil, then reduce to a low simmer. Cook, partially covered, for about 1 hour, until the sauce has reduced. If it boils down too quickly, add a little more water. Taste the sauce and season lightly with pepper (if using).
3. Purée the sauce with a hand-held blender until the required consistency is reached, or the vegetables are completely unnoticeable! Serve with any pasta you like, over meatballs, or even as a sauce for grilled chicken.

Quick Banana Ice Cream

Ingredients
1. 4 ripe bananas
2. 1 tsp vanilla extract

Instructions
1. Simply peel the bananas, chop them into 2cm (¾ in) chunks, and put them in a freezer container. Seal, and put in the freezer until frozen.
2. When the bananas are frozen solid, process them in a food processor with the vanilla extract, until you have a smooth, thick ice cream. You may need to scrape down the sides a couple of times during the process.
3. Either eat the softened banana ice cream immediately, or freeze for a few minutes for it to firm up once more before serving.

Rice Porridge

Ingredients
1. 1 cup dry white rice
2. 4½ cups water
3. ¾ teaspoon salt
4. Optional toppings: fruit, cinnamon, honey

Instructions
1. Add the water to a medium saucepan. Set pan over medium heat until the water reaches a slow boil.
2. In the meantime, use a food processor or coffee grinder to coarsely grind the rice.
3. Add the rice gradually to the boiling water, stirring as you go. When you have added all of the rice to the pan, cover and let simmer for about 4 minutes, until thickened.
4. Serve alone or top with desired toppings.

Brunch Bacon Tortilla

Ingredients
1. 2 tablespoons olive oil
2. 4 unsmoked streaky bacon rashers
3. 6 large eggs425 g (14 oz) potatoes, peeled, cooked and diced
4. 150 g (5 oz) baby tomatoes, halved
5. 1 tablespoon chopped parsley
6. 75 g (3 oz) Cheddar cheese, grated
7. salt and pepper

Instructions
1. Heat 1 tablespoon of the oil in a frying pan over a medium heat, add the bacon and cook for 3–4 minutes. Remove with a slotted spoon.
2. Beat the eggs in a large bowl with some salt and pepper, then stir in the bacon, potatoes, tomatoes and parsley.
3. Heat the remaining oil in the frying pan over a high heat, pour in the egg mixture and cook for 1–2 minutes, then turn down the temperature.
4. Cook for 12–15 minutes, keeping an eye on the edges to make sure the tortilla is not getting too cooked underneath – the top will still be runny.
5. Sprinkle over the grated Cheddar and then place the pan under a preheated hot grill and cook for 3–4 minutes, until golden and bubbling.
6. To turn out, place a plate on top of the pan and turn upside-down.
7. Cut into wedges to serve. This can be eaten hot or cold.

Pigs in Blankets

Ingredients
1. 10 smoked streaky bacon rashers, rind removed
2. 20 pork chipolatas

Instructions
1. Preheat the oven to 200°C (400°F/Gas 6). Take a bacon rasher, place it on a board, and scrape the blade of a knife along it, while pulling on its end, so the bacon stretches out. Cut each piece in half to make 20 short, thin slices.
2. Wrap each chipolata in a half-piece of bacon, then put them on a baking sheet, with the ends of the bacon facing down.
3. Cook in the hot oven for 20–30 minutes, turning occasionally, until the bacon is crispy and the chipolatas cooked through.

Butter Pecan Roasted Sweet Potatoes

Ingredients
1. 6 cups peeled Louisiana yam (sweet potato) cubes (about ½-inch)
2. ¼ cup chopped pecans
3. 2 tablespoons butter, cut into small pieces
4. ⅛ teaspoon cayenne pepper
5. 2 tablespoons light brown sugar

Instructions
1. Preheat oven 400°F. Line baking sheet with foil.

2. Spread cubed sweet potatoes evenly on pan. Bake 30-35 minutes, turning potatoes after 20 minutes.

3. Remove from oven and sprinkle with butter, brown sugar, pecans and cayenne pepper. Return to oven and continue baking 10-15 minutes or until sugar is caramelized.

Chicken & Sweet Potato Soup

Ingredients
1. 2 teaspoons olive oil
2. 1 small onion, chopped
3. 1 garlic clove, crushed
4. 1 red chilli, deseeded and chopped
5. 1 large sweet potato, peeled and cubed
6. 1 large boneless, skinless chicken breast, chopped
7. 1 x 400 g (13 oz) can coconut milk
8. 600 ml (1 pint) chicken stock (see pages 13 and 146)
9. 1 tablespoon chopped fresh coriander
10. salt

Instructions
1. Heat the oil in a nonstick frying pan. Add the onion, garlic and chilli and fry for 3 minutes until softened. Add the sweet potato and chicken and continue to fry for 2–3 minutes until the chicken is coloured all over.

2. Add the coconut milk and stock to the pan, bring to the boil, cover and simmer for 15 minutes until the potato is tender.

3. Transfer to a food processor or blender and process until smooth. Season to taste with salt, stir through the chopped coriander and serve.

Vegan and Vegetarian Crohn's Disease Recipes

Vegan Spelt Plum Cake

Ingredients
1. 1 ¾ ozs coconut oil
2. 1 oz coconut sugar
3. 1 ¾ ozs apple sauce (unsweetened)
4. 3 ½ ozs oat milk
5. 7 ozs
6. spelt- wholemeal flour
7. 2 tsps cream of tartar
8. salt
9. 18 ozs plum

Preparation steps
1. Combine melted coconut oil, coconut blossom sugar, applesauce and oat drink. In a separate bowl, mix whole wheat flour, baking powder and a pinch of salt.
2. Then add flour mixture to the other ingredients and mix well. Pour the batter into a springform pan (greased if necessary).
3. Wash and clean plums, cut in half and remove the core and cut them into wedges. Then spread plums on the batter.
4. Bake vegan plum cake in preheated oven at 180 °C / 350 °F for 40-45 minutes. Then remove from the oven, let cool slightly and serve.

How to Make Vegan Parmesan

Ingredients

1. 5 ¼ ozs cashews
2. 2 tbsps yeast flakes
3. 1 tsp garlic spice
4. salt
5. peppers

Kitchen utensils
1 blender

Preparation steps
1. Place cashews, yeast flakes, garlic seasoning, a pinch of salt and some pepper in a stand mixer and blend for about 30 seconds until a fine consistency is created.
2. Place vegan parmesan in a jar and store it in the refrigerator for up to one week.

Vegan Carbonara

Ingredients
1. 7 ozs cashews
2. 2 tbsps olive oil
3. 4 tbsps yeast flakes
4. 14 ozs vegetable broth
5. salt
6. peppers
7. 14 ozs whole wheat spaghetti
8. 8 ozs tofu
9. 2 garlic cloves
10. 2 tbsps soy sauce
11. 2 tbsps tamari

Preparation steps

1. For the sauce, soak cashews in cold water overnight. The next day, drain, rinse and drain.
2. Place 1 Tablespoon olive oil, cashews, water, yeast flakes, and vegetable broth in a stand blender and puree. Season to taste with salt and pepper.
3. Cook whole grain spaghetti according to package directions in plenty of boiling salted water for 9 - 11 minutes until al dente.
4. Remove smoked tofu from package and dice finely. Peel and finely chop the garlic. Heat 1 tablespoon olive oil in a pan and fry the tofu in it at high temperature for about 2 minutes. Deglaze with soy sauce and tamari sauce and add garlic. Then cook at medium temperature for about 3 minutes. Season to taste with salt and pepper.
5. Pour sauce into a pan and heat. Drain the pasta and mix with the sauce in the pan. Arrange pasta on plates and sprinkle with crispy tofu and optionally serve garnished with some vegan parmesan.

Carrot Hazelnut Cake with cream cheese pistachio icing

Ingredients
1. 14 ozs carrots
2. ½ organic orange
3. 4 eggs
4. 3 ½ ozs raw cane sugar
5. 3 ½ ozs soft butter (and butter for the pan)
6. 7 ozs whole spelt flour
7. 7 ozs ground hazelnuts
8. 2 tsps baking powder

9. 1 pinch salt
10. 7 ozs cream cheese
11. 1 oz shelled pistachio

Preparation steps
1. Clean, wash and finely grate the carrots. Wash orange with hot water, dry, grate 1 tsp. peel and squeeze the juice. Separate eggs and beat egg whites until stiff. Beat sugar with butter and egg yolks until fluffy and fold in 2 Tbsp. orange juice and orange zest.
2. Mix flour, ground hazelnuts, baking powder and salt and add to the butter mixture. Finally, carefully fold in the grated carrots and beaten egg whites.
3. Pour the batter into the greased springform pan and smooth out. Bake in the preheated oven at 180 °C / 350 °F for 60 minutes (test with toothpick), then let cool on a cooling rack.
4. Meanwhile, mix cream cheese with 1 tablespoon orange juice until creamy. Coarsely chop the pistachios. Spread the cooled carrot cake with the cream cheese, sprinkle with pistachios and serve immediately.

Swedish Apple Pie

Ingredients
1. 3 eggs
2. 3 ½ ozs whole cane sugar (+ 1 tablespoon for setting)
3. 5 tbsps spelt- wholemeal flour
4. ½ tsp baking powder
5. 36 ozs sweet apple (e.g. jonagold, granny smiths
6. 1 lemon

7. 1 vanilla bean
8. 2 tbsps cornstarch
9. 3 ½ ozs coconut milk (90% coconut content)

Kitchen utensils
1. 1 springform pan (à 18 cm diameter)

Preparation Step
1. Separate eggs and beat egg whites until stiff. Beat egg yolks and whole cane sugar until foamy. Mix flour and baking powder and gradually stir into the egg-sugar mixture. Carefully fold in egg whites last.
2. Pour the dough into a baking pan (greased if necessary) and bake in a preheated oven at 180 °C / 350 °F for approx. 20 minutes.
3. Meanwhile, wash apples and dry them. Peel and grate coarsely with a grater. Squeeze lemon juice and pour over apples.
4. Cut vanilla bean in half lengthwise and scrape out vanilla pulp with a knife. Mix cornstarch with 1 tablespoon whole cane sugar. Put 7 ounces of water in a saucepan. Add sugar-starch mixture to the pot and stir to dissolve. Then stir in vanilla pulp and cinnamon.
5. Mix the finished mixture with the grated apples and spread on the cooled cake base. Refrigerate for about 2 hours.
6. When the cake is completely cooled, whip coconut milk and spread on the cake. Optional: dust pie with a little cinnamon, then cut into pieces and serve.

Low Carb Brownies with Apricots

Ingredients
1. 3 ½ ozs soft butter (+ some for the pan)
2. 2 ozs maple syrup
3. 1 tsp vanilla extract
4. 4 eggs
5. 7 ozs almond flour
6. 3 tbsps cocoa powder (highly deoiled)
7. 2 tsps baking powder
8. 1 pinch salt
9. 4 tbsps milk (whole)
10. 3 ½ ozs dark chocolate (min. 70% cocoa content)
11. 7 ozs apricot

Kitchen utensils
1. 1 hand mixer, 1 bowl, 1 loaf pan (20 x 30 cm)

Preparation Step
1. Beat butter, maple syrup, vanilla extract and eggs in a bowl until fluffy.
2. Mix almond flour, cocoa powder, baking powder and salt in a bowl. Melt dark chocolate over a water bath or in the microwave.
3. Mix the dry ingredients and liquid ingredients alternately with the milk and chocolate until smooth. Pour the mixture into a greased baking pan. Wash the apricots and pat them dry. Cut in half, remove the stone, and cut into quarters. Spread apricots on top of the brownie mixture and bake in a preheated oven at 180 °C / 350 ° F for 20 minutes.

Tofu Fingers with Lime Dip

Ingredients
1. 14 ozs firm tofu
2. 7 ozs whole grain breadcrumbs
3. 1 tsp sweet paprika
4. 1 tbsp olive oil
5. salt
6. peppers
7. 4 tbsps cornstarch
8. 5 ozs soy milk
9. 1 organic lime
10. ½ bunch parsley
11. 7 ozs soy yogurt
12. 1 pinch cayenne pepper

Preparation steps
1. Drain tofu and cut into 1-inch thick strips. In a bowl, mix whole grain bread crumbs, paprika powder, olive oil, salt, and pepper. Put cornstarch and soy milk in bowls respectively.
2. Roll the tofu strips first in starch, then in soy milk and then in the breadcrumb mixture. Place the strips on a baking tray lined with baking paper and bake in a preheated oven at 180°C / 350°F for 10 minutes until crispy.
3. For the dip, rinse lime, dry, and then grate the zest and squeeze juice from half the lime. Wash parsley, shake dry, and chop finely. Place soy yogurt in a bowl and mix with parsley, salt, cayenne pepper, lime juice, and zest.
4. Remove the tofu sticks from the oven and serve with the dip.

Pumpkin and Tomato Bowl

Ingredients
1. 1 small hokkaido pumpkin (20-22 ounces)
2. 1 red onion
3. 1 garlic clove
4. 9 ozs cherry tomatoes
5. 9 ozs chickpeas (can; drained weight)
6. 2 tbsps olive oil
7. 3 ½ ozs soy creamer
8. salt
9. peppers
10. ½ tsp cumin
11. 1 pinch red pepper flakes
12. 1 handful parsley

Preparation steps
1. Clean the pumpkin, wash, halve, remove the core and cut the pumpkin flesh into slices. Peel, halve and slice the onion. Peel and chop garlic. Wash tomatoes and cut in half lengthwise. Rinse chickpeas and drain.
2. Heat oil in a frying pan and sauté onion, garlic and pumpkin for 5 minutes over medium heat.
3. Then add chickpeas and tomatoes and steam for another 5 minutes. Add soy cream, bring to the boil briefly and season with salt, pepper, cumin and chili flakes. Wash parsley, shake dry and chop. Serve chickpea-tomato pan sprinkled with parsley.

Chickpea and Pumpkin Pasta

Ingredients
1. 30 ozs whole grain pasta (spirelli)
2. salt
3. 10 ozs hokkaido pumpkin pulp (or butternut squash
4. 1 red onion
5. 8 ozs cherry tomatoes
6. 9 ozs chickpeas (can; drained weight)
7. 2 tbsps olive oil
8. 5 ozs oat cream
9. peppers
10. 1 pinch red pepper flakes
11. 1 handful parsley

Preparation steps
1. Cook pasta according to package directions in plenty of boiling salted water for about 9-10 minutes until al dente, drain in a colander and drain.
2. Along the way, cut pumpkin pulp into slices. Peel, halve and slice the onion. Wash tomatoes and cut in half lengthwise. Rinse chickpeas and drain.
3. Heat oil in a frying pan, sauté onion, and pumpkin for 5 minutes over medium heat. Then add chickpeas and saute for another 5 minutes. Add oat milk, about 4-6 Tbsp water, and bring to a boil. Season with salt, pepper, and chili flakes.
4. Wash the parsley, shake dry and chop. Arrange the pasta with the chickpeas and tomatoes on plates and serve the autumnal pasta sprinkled with parsley.

Vegan Blueberry Muffins

Ingredients
1. 1 ¾ ozs raw cane sugar
2. 1 ¾ ozs sugar free apple sauce
3. 9 ozs oat milk
4. 3 ½ tbsps canola oil
5. 1 vanilla bean (or 2 tsp vanilla extract)
6. 6 ozs whole spelt flour
7. 3 ½ ozs oats
8. 2 tsps cream of tartar
9. salt
10. 6 ozs blueberries

Kitchen utensils
1. 1 muffin tin

Preparation steps
1. Mix raw cane sugar with applesauce, oat milk, and canola oil. Cut vanilla bean in half lengthwise, scrape out vanilla pulp with a knife and stir in. Mix spelt flour with oat flakes, baking powder, and a pinch of salt. Add to the remaining ingredients, mix everything into a smooth dough.
2. Wash and sort the blueberries, then carefully fold into the batter. Pour the batter into a muffin tin lined with muffin cups and bake in a preheated oven at 180 °C / 350 °F for about 25 minutes until golden brown.
3. Remove vegan blueberry muffins from oven, let cool briefly and serve.

CONCLUSION

Flare-ups of Crohn's can cause diarrhea, abdominal pain, and loss of appetite. If symptoms persist, they can lead to malnutrition and dehydration.

During a flare-up, it is best to drink plenty of fluids and avoid foods that aggravate symptoms. Eating foods that are easy to digest and rich in nutrients can help ease symptoms and promote healing.

During remission, it is important to eat a balanced, nutritious diet. It may be best to speak with a doctor or dietitian before making any significant dietary changes.

www.ingramcontent.com/pod-product-compliance
Lightning Source LLC
Chambersburg PA
CBHW050742260726
48661CB00001B/371